Health - What is yours, and what belongs to your family system

Seeing how mapping the health of our history can help us be really healthy

Rafe Nauen ©2018

Contents

Copyright

ISBN-13: 978-1518895586

ISBN-10: 1518895581

Foreword

If you do what you've always done, then you'll get what you've always got! Change exists with stretch and this book is about mapping the change potential within your life and that of your family and hence breaking cycles or repeated patterns

This book is to allay any fears that might surround looking at a family system in a group setting.

With many coaching models the boundary one often reaches (and sometimes rather quickly) is that solutions to the issues are not sitting in the room, be they structures, history, perhaps family, ancestry or even ethics.

With the model described herein that boundary evaporates, because the system is looked at as a whole with the individual players in that system finding the best place for themselves. Surprisingly, or perhaps unsurprisingly, when one person finds exactly the right place, others and sometimes all the others find a better, or even the right place within the system. No-one quite has the answer to how, or why – it just seems to work like that.

Introduction

I got into constellation work as a result of needing personal counselling in connection with the imminent death of my then wife Maia. The psychotherapist Isaac Pizer introduced me to constellations therapy almost straight away and I was blown away. It showed that I could see what I was carrying in my life, what belonged to me and what didn't. That story is described more fully in my first book *Family Constellations – Unravelling the mystery of your ancestral timeline.*

I have had a number of career channels in my life thus far and constellations work seemed to fit exactly with what I wanted to do next. Studying constellations theory and practice over two years brought up the fact that constellations (so called because the apparent connection between constellations in the sky is not by any physical means – they just appear to be grouped thus, in other words, because they are!) And so it is with businesses or families, or indeed with any grouping that could be called a system.

I find that many systems would welcome a virtual map of the influences and people inside and outside those systems especially if it were simple and not require any prior adaptions or changes. Here is the answer to that particular prayer. The term constellations always needs a description, but in the Germanic countries where this work mostly hails from, it is widely known.

Some of this book requires acceptance that feelings a) exist and b) are important in all matters. If you doubt that, ask someone to make 20 cold calls on a Friday afternoon. I assure you that if they don't feel like it – they will find a way for it not to happen – something more important might well come up in that scenario.

When faced with group work – and although this method works extremely well on a one to one situation, a workshop is where this stuff flies – many people feel or expect to feel intimidated and anxious – will they be able to express themselves correctly – what level of participation can they manage etc. etc. This book is to allay at least some of those fears. You may wish to read my first book *Family Constellations – Unravelling the mystery of your ancestral timeline.*

One additional aspect has revealed itself during my work in this field. Healing and Curing are not one and the same thing. It is definitely possible to achieve either one without the other. At the end of the day we will all die and we will no doubt die **of** something. Super Hospitals are definitely a curing place. If they get to know what is wrong, they are exceptionally good at rectifying the problem. But we live in an age of fear, where a nurse fears cuddling an upset patient in case it should be misinterpreted in some sexual or abusive way. Thus the hospital has moved away from giving a healing experience and has concentrated on the curing principles. Many people believe that food cooked with care and love has some healing qualities – old Jewish traditions using chicken soup are a case in point. Thus a hospital that doesn't even cook food (microwaved cook-chill foods coming from a factory), let alone cooking it with care and love maybe missing a trick in its art-form. It has been shown that people get better quicker (cure faster) in a healing environment.

In view of the fact that 100% of all people who either go to hospital or who don't, will, in due course, die, then the medical profession's quest to always find a cure and to regard it as a failure in the event of not doing so (success rates in hospital?) will always fail in the long run. So it is the short run that is concentrated on with the emphasis on getting people fixed up to return to the fray of the life they led before. The concept of providing health care – to preserve life at any cost, becomes a) futile and b) destined to run over budget!

In the realm of mental health care, there is a multitude of evidence that people are treated for the short term and often merely to remove them from the here and now for the other people – the doctor or the family. To subdue. Many anti-psychotic drugs have a multiplicity of side effect symptoms, which often include the issue for which they were prescribed in the first place. Getting someone fixed up and out of here is the primary objective. To open the can of worms the lies beneath has huge penalties for the practitioner for fear that the lid will be impossible to replace. However, seen in terms of multigenerational trauma (see chapter 4 for an explanation), perhaps there is much more long term healing work needing to be done, especially in understanding the consequences of one generations attitudes and actions on another and subsequent generations. It would be unusual in the medical world we find ourselves in 2018 to start looking at what happened to a patient's grandfather during the last war, as an aide to recovery for the patient today. However, my limited research would tend to support such a move.

Acknowledgements

Isaac Pizer, who started the ball rolling with me in the world of constellations, and who remains my supervisor, Richard Wallstein who introduced me to the work, and remains a much respected colleague, Stephan Hausner whose book "Even if it costs me my life" inspired me to look, and also introduced me to the concept of MSP (Chapter 5). My wife Julie Bowman who has encouraged me, and my family who I have observed and who have in turn inspired me.

Chapter 1 - What is a constellation?

So, what is a constellation (apart from a group of stars) – well fundamentally, it's a living map that reveals the hidden dynamics of any system. A system is any group defined by the relationship they have to each other – family, workgroup, board of directors and so on. In this book, I am concentrating on health, but the rules apply to any grouping of people or things that might be regarded as a system – even down to a chronic illness – that will be discussed later, but by way of example someone has a painful broken leg. Clearly the problem is in the leg, or perhaps they are even more precise and say their knee is the issue, but their lack of mobility will have a profound effect on what they are able to do. They might have suffered some severe trauma getting the damaged knee, so could have nightmares, quite apart from the normal sleep deprivation from pain. That may mean that they get annoyed or upset more than would be normal for them. The family then will have to rally round – transport, maybe the bedroom is inaccessible so things will change in the house and maybe there is a sudden drop in income that coincides with a sudden increase in costs, so worry in the family will increase. They may be concerned that a parent or grandparent had a tumour in their knee and this is a recurrence. They may start being secretive in the hope of "protecting" their family from the awful possibility that they have a similar fate looming to Grandpa Albert. They may have emotional side effects from the pain killers and prescription drugs they have been advised to take. And so on. So you can see that looking at basic elements on their own is a far from perfect way to arrive at successful outcomes and sometimes it can be far more useful to look at the system.

The starting point is always someone who wants to look at an issue, perhaps there's a recurrent problem at work, or some situation that they can't quite come to grips with. It may be a forced change within the system – a death, a birth, a marriage or a divorce, or "problems" with a child's behaviour may becoming noticeably difficult to deal with, or in this book, you have noticed that your health reveals a pattern, or a metaphor that suggests the cause may not be immediately within your grasp and thus neither will be the solution. Constellations are a powerful way of working with such issues. Rather than look at the individual or the place where the problem is, we look at the whole system, however widely that forces us to look. That's because an individual is always part of a much wider interconnected system and the problem may just be a symptom of something that's actually happening elsewhere. That was exactly true in my case and I shall be using my own experience as well as other people's whose constellations I have facilitated further on in this book.

What we do is set up a visual spatial representation of that system. Ideally we use people to represent the different parts of the system so it becomes a living map or constellation, but pieces of felt on a floor, post it notes or even PlayPeople™[1] can be used. We then ask those representatives to listen to their feelings, their sensations and their intuitions and what happens is that the underlying dynamics of the system come to the surface. It seems that simply the client giving permission for an element of their existence to be represented is enough for the display of the dynamics to begin. Many hundreds of thousands of workshops have been noted and written up and they all show that some hidden dynamics have been revealed that have hitherto lain hidden.

---

[1] Playpeople are sold as toys, but also in sets for constellation practitioners. They are used as representatives – especially of the juxtaposition between people in families, and are exceptionally good at enabling children to articulate deep psychological issues with families, abuse or with health.

Constellations rely on some underlying principles - a bit like a house relies on gravity.

1. Everyone has an equal right to belong - everyone who enters a system (a new baby for example) has a right to as much love as anyone else and it can be shown that having "favourites" causes issues down the line

2. Things that come before have to give way to things that come later - an older sibling has to allow his or her world to change a little for the survival of the system and his or her place within it, irrespective of the trauma it may cause to the older sibling.

3. Systems that come later take precedence over older systems. If someone has a child in the context of an affair, it can be pretty harsh for the original family system. The person who has partially moved away and into a new system, will have much more energy for the new system, whatever they say to themselves, or whatever promises they may make. Ironically this may be even truer if the new system is denied.

4. The balance of giving and receiving needs to be maintained - common sense (and a great deal of research) has shown that balance must be maintained in all things, especially family systems.

My style as a constellation facilitator is to sit in a circle of potential clients or issue holders and to ask and see who is willing or best placed to start working on an issue. There is a clear moment when someone has made the decision that the pain of maintaining their trauma or bonding dilemma is outweighed by the tantalising hope of a good outcome and a resolution so that the next phase of life begins without their old misplaced associations. If the facilitator is skilled, noticing that moment is of huge benefit, as the energy the client then brings to the work is significantly enhanced. It also drives responsibility to its rightful place, as the client is entirely in control of the process and simply needs some affirmations or confirmations as to the way the method then enables the unfolding of their own story and uncovering of misplaced dramas or traumas. The client may decide that the price is too high and that in actual fact they would prefer to live with what they know rather than perhaps expose secrets to the glare of the truth. It is a) their choice, but b) also of itself very empowering as they still remain in control of the process. For the facilitator that interferes – for example he or she may have already decided who will work and in what order, can him or herself become a representative of an overbearing or instructive element within the client's family system, unknowingly and thereby create an entanglement that adds to the client's woes, rather than diminish them. It may also completely hide the real issue from the work.

I often will enquire how the client themselves are doing to check that a) nothing is unravelling in a different way to that showing up and b) that the client is not getting too much and would rather leave it for now and return to the subject at a later date. I will probably encourage sticking with it and often a distressed client will be asked "yes, but can you manage?". Sometimes within a constellation workshop, a representative will mention a smell or feeling that relates directly to the clients own feelings or smell associations. That of itself may unlock a doorway or portal to another dimension of the work and yield a whole layer of data that until that moment remained hidden. For me, as a facilitator, those moments have to treated with great respect and care, as an example will illustrate. One client had set up a constellation with her mother, her father and herself. Grief had appeared and it turned out that this related to the death of a sibling. I asked someone to enter the constellation as a representative of the dead child. The mother broke down in tears and it showed some disquiet in the father, although it didn't look like grief.

However, this seemed to be enough story and I just needed to let the constellation run its course, perhaps suggest some rituals for the excessively late bereavement (over 40 years) of the sibling on behalf of the mother. But then the representative revealed that she could smell rotting meat. Observation of the client (at that time sitting out and watching) showed a distinct change of pallor, countenance and agitation. I enquired in my usual style – "What's going on?" she then revealed a long history of sexual abuse and an eating disorder that meant that meat was distinctly repulsive to her. Her father – the abuser – had insisted on her eating the meat, so she had taken it to her room and hidden it. The resulting smell unlocked the whole sorry saga. The father's representative went through a whole array of feelings from anger, shame, rejection and included wanting to leave (sometimes this reveals suicidal tendencies) and it explained something I had noticed, but had done nothing about – why the father had been unable to look at the mother and seemed bonded to the daughter (the client issue holder). Allowing the smell to be a facet of the work in that case unlocked the real reason for the client attending such a workshop. Her shame had held her with secrets, but the smell noticed by the representative unlocked the doorway for the client, gave her confidence that the constellation was genuinely looking at her stuff and wasn't made up! The moment of the price being too high had passed!

Chapter 3 – The study of health using constellations

When I work with clients, either in one to one sessions, or in workshops, I notice that new things come up, maybe metaphors such as pains in the back registering with an unsupported feeling or a perpetual stomach pain associated with inability to stomach issues within the family etc. etc. I notice somatic symptoms – where there is a symptom in the body that clearly derives from an emotional pain. Having gathered new data from the experiential reporting from the client, I then make connections with research or other writers on the subject and new insights emerge. Then when I am next working with a client I find other levels of awareness start to arise.

The beauty of the constellations model is that the client and I are working in tandem and as it is not a talking therapy the danger of implanting thoughts is very limited and gives immense freedom to the process. At no time do I become superior in any way within the client's system. In counselling, it is quite common for a client to justify an action or remark by saying, "My therapist …." That shouldn't ever happen in a constellation because what is revealed is revealed by a) the permission of the client to look and b) the noticing by the representatives. The facilitator may enable some experiments – it may show up what looks like the death of a child within a constellation, so I will add a representative for that secret, but if nothing changes in the other representatives, then I abandon the idea as an experiment whose validity is the same in success as in failure. The addition of the child in the example above added a whole new dimension.

Chapter 4 – Trauma

People experience trauma in different ways, and the body has different mechanisms to deal with it. For example a bad road accident where you get trapped and lose a leg, the body will kick in with survival techniques at the time, and you may feel numb, or no pain and then later, when your brain has decided that you can deal with it the pain kicks in.

When the trauma is only witnessed the body has no such systems because the trauma experienced is linked to the connection or the empathy. So, Ambulance driver, Paramedic, the victim, any witnesses and the family of the victim, and perhaps the car driver who escaped free but actually caused the collision in the first place, and indeed his or her family, can all experience different kinds of trauma, and have very different responses to it as well.

Chapter 5 - MSP – Multigenerational Systemic Psychotraumatology

I usually try to avoid jargon, especially in a book such as this, aimed at clients who have not even come across the word constellations in this context let alone "Multigenerational Systemic Psychotraumatology". Well, sometimes avoiding jargon requires repeated long sentences of explanation. And here, MSP describes very eloquently an everyday, but often missed issue. "Trauma experienced in a mother will be expressed and experienced by the children". This as a general principle, holds up well. It is likely the mother embedded in the principle will over protect, to avoid the reoccurrence, under protect and pass on in loyalty to the older system, or do some work on herself to alleviate the symptoms of her trauma. At no stage however, will it simply have gone away. It will be around, although perhaps in a changed format. Sometimes we exchange sensations in the emotional world with feelings in the physical realm, or in the mental. But the principle stands and applies not just to mothers. MSP (Multigenerational Systemic Psychotraumatology) is the study of the way we handle trauma within different generations in family systems and is the fundamental basis for looking at health in families using the constellation model.

It is trauma in one generation that creates experiences that make us wish to freeze or flee inappropriately and set up chains of events that if we are unable to reconcile, manage or actually deal with, we will automatically pass on to the next generation.

Sometimes the trauma is (on the memory level at least) unknown. In those circumstances, the constellation model is pretty adept at revealing it.

The classic example of MSP that anyone can relate to, and which has some considerable scientific research is from the survivors of Auschwitz. Many people at a concentration camp wanted to die even sooner than they were being enabled to die. Failure to commit suicide and "save" themselves and their children can leave an element in the family where someone might feel that death is a saving grace. In the UK every year there are 200 filicides (that's killing your own children). Factor in what happened prior to their situation and you might find an explanation that just about explains that particular mindset.

Constellations would enable the visiting of that particular scenario prior to it being played out in real life, and might lead to someone appreciating the fact that killing your children will not save them, especially outside a concentration camp.

How?

I refer you back to Chapter 1 which explains what happens. No-one is quite sure how or even why, but from the extensive research and reporting there is no doubt that we carry information that was not created during our lifetime. It was born with us. Some of it is pretty obvious if you look at things a bit differently.

Mum and Dad have a still born child – mum is devastated. Dad hasn't begun to bond with the child. The mourn, vow not to let it get them down, decide not to talk about it, and have another child. The second child. But brought up in the place of the first – more often than you would expect, with the name the first child was to have been given.

In this scenario, it is hard to imagine it having anything less than a huge impact on all the subsequent family system.

Chapter 6 – The mechanics of a workshop

What happens in a constellation workshop? I am going to use a real example from a workshop held some years ago

Who is in a constellation?

The facilitator; someone who guides the process, but who remains as far as possible, outside the process

A seeker; someone who feels the urge to look at their stuff, right now – they will probably be a bit fired up, enthusiastic – their moment has arrived.

Representatives; people who will get asked to represent other people during the process – placeholders certainly, but sometimes quite a bit more

Participants; the rest of the people in the workshop – they sit around the edge of the working area and hold the energy – they just observe mostly – they will get a chance to be a seeker, or a participant later

Only the facilitator will necessarily have had prior experience of constellation work, but some, maybe all of the others will have attended workshops before – even participants get a big learning from the work.

Everyone sits around in a circle of chairs – preferably about 18-20 feet across the circle. The facilitator will have picked a place to sit and have a vacant chair next to him or her. He or she will probably do a short meditation, so that everyone is calm, relaxed and body conscious – by that I mean that people become aware of what is going on in their own body, so that they can express changes that occur – these may become quite important as the work progresses. The circle inside the chairs is called the field – like a field of energy and is identified to establish boundaries to the work.

Firstly, a seeker is chosen. The facilitator may choose, or ask who is ready, or maybe another method is used. The seeker comes and sits by the facilitator. For this example, let's say the seeker is female and forty-six years old and the facilitator is me! This movement symbolises moving into a place where other things become enabled. The seeker then tells the facilitator the facts. The facilitator is not interested in blame, or opinion, just facts – such as my mother and father are still alive; they separated when I was two and I haven't seen my father since that day; my mother had two miscarriages before I was born, but I have an older brother that survived. My mother remarried when I was two and a half.

What the facilitator is doing here is to identify the important elements in what was around during the seekers early life – more importance is placed on things that happened in the family before the seeker was born, because those things will have moulded the seeker. The facilitator will no doubt make a judgement call on whether to set up the mother's new husband at the outset, or to see if he figures later. Again, a judgement call will be required to reckon whether the miscarriages are significant – sometimes they are and sometimes they aren't. In this work, we find that abortions always have a place, still births always have a place and miscarriages do only sometimes.

So I ask the seeker what is her burning desire (or some such form of words) – this enables an intention to be set and is useful but not essential to the work. She says "All my relationships die too soon". She says she has a mother (still alive) a father (still alive) and an elder brother. She thinks her mother had a miscarriage between her brother and her. I ask her to choose four people to represent herself, her mother, her father and her brother. I choose not to complicate matters just yet by requesting a representative of the miscarried baby. It is simpler for me to work if the representatives are women for women and men for men, but in truth it is not important. I have run several constellations where there were a lot of one sex and insufficient of the other for that rule to apply. A basic fundamental of the work is "Working with what is" – in other words we all have to survive and succeed with whatever deal of cards we get – we can make the best of it, just as easily as the worst of it. I know a woman whose father was a real bully. He terrorised her but she learned to stick out her jaw and say "Yeah, that all you got?" many years later she was on the front line at Greenham Common when an American soldier pointed a machine gun at her. She was part of thousands of women campaigning to not have American missiles launched from English soil without our involvement in a war. She stuck out her jaw and suggested "Go on then, pull the trigger if you've got the balls" Of course he backed down. She had learned to resource herself from her terrible experiences as a child.

So what happens next? I ask her to set the representatives up – by which I mean she asks them if they are willing to act as a representative. If they say yes, they stand up and she stands behind them with hands lightly on their shoulders and she moves them to a place in the field (the space within the circle of chairs) that "feels right". Extraordinarily, whilst it sounds odd, there is such a place and so far no-one in a workshop has ever struggled to find such a place!

So now we have four people standing up, in the circle and the seeker now sits down to watch, to listen and to feel. She cannot interrupt, or even interject – but I may ask confirmation of things that I see, or for more information when something odd crops up.

The seeker's rep is standing alone in the middle, the father is standing near the edge looking out, the mother is near the edge looking in, towards the father and the brother is near the middle, again looking towards the father. So what can I work on? Let's make some assumptions. One of the beauties of this work is that we can test hypotheses readily and easily without any ecological damage (i.e. we can experiment without any problems occurring further down the line). I suggest that dad would rather be somewhere else (in constellation speak, he wishes to leave) Dad relaxes immediately and even moves to do just that, leave. I ask him where his interest lies – he says comrades. I ask the seeker if she has any idea what this means, because it means nothing to me, nor to the participants and representatives present at this workshop, not even the representative that uttered the word!

She says "my dad worked on a minesweeper in the war and he was called away for some important work on another ship and whilst he was gone his ship went down with all hands on deck. He was devastated and felt he should have died with his comrades"

I ask three people to stand just outside the circle near the dad, to represent the comrades who died. They seem happy and not troubled, which surprises all of us, especially dad! I ask him to talk to them and for them to respond. A dialogue ensues where it becomes clear that dad surviving felt good to the others – he got a life, a beautiful daughter and for him to have died would have stopped that and that would have been in no-one's interest.

So what's going on here? People who have never met, are having a conversation that they could never have had and would never happen in reality. It displays a general attitude to death and has a distinct relationship with understanding and relieving survivor guilt. And that element of the situation wasn't even known at the outset, so how did dad's representative come up with "Comrades"?

It seems that we carry with us a metaphysical energy that contains truths and aspects that protect us and keep us safe in our journey. Sometimes the trauma surrounding such things becomes outmoded and can safely be dropped. When we "set people up" in a constellation we are handing over permission for a small part of that energy to be replicated within a virtual map and gives us the ability to observe and to change those energies.

Humans are unusual in that nearly everything they take into later life is borne out of a loyalty to parenting – maybe not actual father and mother, but the process of parenting which means that children learn to become adults and eventually become adults with whatever they have picked up along the way.

I have noticed that dad's representative is wanting to turn towards the field – I suggest he follows that movement and I can see that he is looking warmer. I suggest some words he might say. This is a facilitator technique for uncovering some historical truths. We can suggest words and then when they have said, ask the person who said them to say if they felt true. Surprisingly, they will probably have a strong feeling either way – very seldom an "I'm not sure" In this case I ask him to say to his daughter "I didn't know you were there" the seekers rep bursts into tears. He offers a hug and they hold an embrace for a while. The other reps have turned to look and the brother's rep is crying a little too. Mum look radiant.

In this short exercise, it has become clear that the most important perceived relationship for the father was to his dead comrades and thus it becomes clear that the daughter – our seeker here, has spent her life so far looking for relationships that become dead out of love for her dad and that to have been associated with life and vibrancy would have been disloyal. Clearly this is errant nonsense. However, what has happened here is that everything has changed in a short space of time. The representatives are thanked and they sit down. I suggest that chatter is minimal and that discussion about who did what to who and why should be let go of. The work has begun, but has not yet ended. The seeker now has to allow the change to permeate her body and mind, such that every cell has a very slightly different outlook. That can take time and is best done with space and not clamour. I also suggest that for confidentiality reasons that any discussion of the works should definitely include this piece of work, but with enough detail removed or changed to protect identities completely – just as I have in this book.

So feedback from this particular piece of work – the seeker can have a relationship with someone who wishes very much to be alive and for the relationship itself to be alive. The mother has seen what she intrinsically knew was there already and the son has been seen and can now model himself on a father that wishes to be present. And the father can breathe again! Instead of feeling every day that he should have died with his comrades – the message to his daughter gets to feel like it would have been more correct if she had not been born – hardly a healthy paradigm to live under!

There is an underlying truth with the loyalty thing. If you are a man, you should ideally be a bit like your dad and marry someone a bit like your mum. Equally, if you are a woman you should be a bit like your mum and marry someone a bit like your dad. In many cases that is observable fact and I have even observed a gay man whose partner was quite a bit like his mum in attitudes and personality even. If you look around, it is common enough for this to be true!

Chapter 7 – What health conditions can we constellate?

The simple answer is anything that has connection to a system can be constellated. Generally chronic conditions are the most likely to have some MSP aspects that can be shifted or alleviated using the constellations method. Mental conditions can be very effectively examined, but in these cases, (as in all cases and indeed in all psychotherapeutic work) it is always worth checking what would happen to the client if the condition was eradicated permanently. Often the condition performs several functions within a system and an ecological check-up is always essential.

To be definitive for a moment:

1. Weight disorders – obesity/anorexia/bulimia
2. Crone's disease
3. Back pain
4. Skin conditions
5. IBS
6. Cancer
7. Addictions
   a. Alcohol
   b. Smoking
   c. Gambling
8. Sleep apnoea
9. Panic attacks

10. Depression
11. Bipolar disorder (Manic Depression)
12. Borderline Personality Disorder (BPD)

This is not a definitive list, but a guideline to the sort of conditions that might be worthy of a look. If medication is involved, then the client must always take responsibility for engaging with the doctor to establish if reduction or cessation of medical treatment would be advantageous. A Constellation facilitator should never recommend a course, or the cessation of a course of medicines prescribed by a medical professional.

In one constellation a woman had had a skin condition for years, but had recently realised that her father had a skin condition and his attitude to her had been appalling and that metaphorically he made her skin crawl (her words). The constellation shows the relationship to be more than coincidence. So she sets up the work to show what a skin condition might do for her and who it really belonged to. It showed that the story went back and back and that the resolution involved ritual sending back of things that no longer or never did belong.

Constellations provide an easy platform for certain types of ritual. In this case getting the fathers representative to state that "This has nothing to do with you, you are just a child" and his father's representative to say the same and his father's representative to say the same along a line of people in the workshop, just seems to be enough. In this case the work had become possible after the woman's father's death.

Prior to that, the price of having that dialogue would have been too high – we might say she wasn't ready, but to engage with the father only as an ancestor enabled the work to flow and meant that dealing with his abuse and violence during her childhood was comparatively simple.

Chapter 8 – Suicide

In many families, there will have been suicides in the past. Often not spoken about and often shrouded in shame and guilt.

Children are designed to be loyal to family systems – if you are a man, you are supposed to be a bit like your dad, and marry someone a bit like your mum. If you are a woman, be a bit like your mum and marry someone a bit like your dad. I have worked with gay men that bear that out, even though the gender of their husband was different. The reason is that the species of mankind is designed to adapt to change, but to keep the development gradual and as slow as possible.

So, if a family member died young, or in terrible circumstances, there might be a residue of pressure within the family system for someone later to balance that energy by dying early. Getting someone who shows signs of feeling like that to a constellation can have a remarkable effect – they may feel angry, because that route of escape is now blocked, but they remain alive where the issue can be resolved over time, and prevent the energy of that issue remaining within the system, and remaining unresolved, so that someone later will need to create that balance.

Chapter 10 – Cancer

Cancer has a special place in health. Mostly people feel that a cancer diagnosis is a death sentence. Survival rates are getting better, but an understanding of the disease is important.

The brain sends out "kill" signals all the time to cells in the body. The average cell at the outside edge of a finger lasts about 3 weeks. The cornea lasts a lifetime. Few cells survive beyond 7 years. The "kill" signals are designed to ensure new cells develop and grow and keep the body healthy. Mostly the cells respond to the kill signal by dying and being absorbed if internal, or rubbing off if external. However when a part becomes unhealthy, it may not respond the signal, and "refuses" to die. The part then gets involved in cell division itself (the normal healing process which is in all of us all the time) and a tumour develops.

When we define someone's cancer diagnosis, the question most often asked is "Where has he or she got it?" the answer is entirely up to you. "In a cell in my leg", "in a tumour in my leg", "in my leg", "in me", "in my family", and so on. They are all true.

How can a constellation help with cancer?

You will discover where the cancer belongs in the system, because frequently it is not exactly in the patient. They may be someone who often says, "I'll do it for you" and in those circumstances they may be unable to avoid the outcome. They may feel that if they pass the health issue "back" they will be guilty of hurting someone else – a price too high. However, they may realize that they are not doing that, they are balancing the system, and that when everything is where it should be, even if that means talking about some things that family feel would be better left as a secret, they will automatically be healthier.

Chapter 11 – Eating Disorders

Eating disorders are very often engaged to hide something. There has been considerable research into anorexia and invariably the sufferer feels themselves much larger than the tape measure shows them to be. This confusion often arises from sexual abuse from within a family system – mixed messages by the perpetrator and by the others in the system – maybe complicit maybe also abused and maybe absent for their own reasons. The bonding of the mother to the father may significantly change on the birth of the child and the father may feel rejected and abandoned – reminiscent of his own childhood perhaps. The search for intimacy then drives him to fail to honour proper boundaries and the system becomes abused. The daughter becomes anorexic as part of a pattern of confusion of trust and of failing to understand her place in any sense.

In one of my clients I found that several stepdaughters had been sexually abused from a very early age. The one that suffered from eating disorders had actually not been sexually abused at all. She was completely aware of the other sister's abuse and felt she wasn't pretty enough to attract the abuser. In some ways her abuse was the more difficult to reconcile.

Talking to such an example of historic anorexia in terms of nutrition and healthy eating can be seen as well beyond pointless. The fact of her appearance and the notion of her appearance are forever in different places and until those two aspects have been associated and reconciled nothing will change.

Sometimes the eating disorder is a survival strategy to alleviate the hidden knowledge of the untimely death of an ancestral relative. In past generations – say before the 1700s it was common to lose children in childbirth and mourning was routine and ritualised commonly. Many mothers died in childbirth and many communities had standard methods for handling such affairs. Sometimes a sibling's family semi-automatically took on the dead mother's children. Then in the Georgian and Victorian eras shame and guilt became a tool for managing communities and much of that ritual disappeared. An unwritten code of silence was implanted and when a still birth happened, no-one spoke of it. Indeed, sometimes the next surviving child was even given the name of the deceased child. If you agree that naming of children is usually to mimic our heroes by association (there are very few Adolfs christened since WWII) then naming a child after a child that died in birth is a risky thing to do (NB in my book on Family Constellation I recount the story of my brother's experience to that end). Fast forward a generation or two and the pressure to survive against all odds might readily yield itself to the field. In that scenario a person might feel they need to eat anything that becomes available, to ensure good health, including survival of the species. In year 10,000 BC living off fruit and squirrels whilst living in a wood, the eating disorder suggested by that scenario might not show itself very clearly, but in 2015, with incredible availability of food obesity comes very easily. We don't have to exercise and we can eat anything. Whilst I am not suggesting that all obesity comes from a grandmother that had a still born child, I am suggesting that it is one of the precursors, in the same way that anorexia has been shown to often occur in families where sexual abuse of the child has occurred. In young children, sexual abuse, especially by a parent, usually the father or stepfather is exceptionally confusing. They feel wrong yet loved or special (they may well have been groomed into that situation) they feel adult yet still a child, nurtured and abused all at the same time, so for them to come out with a confusion about what they feel, as opposed to what they see in the mirror is hardly surprising. Note the reference above to the girl who became anorexic because she herself felt that she hadn't been pretty enough to get the attention of the abuser.

Chapter 12 – How to set up a constellation about health

Experience and judgement and gut instinct give us the start point, which seldom matters, as the constellation method is very adept at sowing us the way forward. When there are gaps, they show up, when there are unusual connections and associations, they show up and when we get it wrong and need to work a different way it shows up – maybe in the form that there is just no energy in the room to work with, or it feels as if there is no permission.

People or aspects? We can set up constellations with either or both. If the client has a propensity to hypochondria when we might start by assuming that the illnesses perceived perform some supportive role in the system. That assumption might be shown to be correct or incorrect in the initial work. We work with what is and set up the participants that have "shown up" in the conversation, so our initial setup might include the client, the illness, the mother and the intent for example. The facilitator will always need to choose whether the client represents themselves, or whether he or she is represented by a participant.

Sometimes the free movement of participants will show the direction of flow towards a better or ideal outcome, sometimes, a bit of guidance is required, with some dialogue between the facilitator and the representatives in question. If you can imagine a scenario where an illness almost has a personality, the constellation method gives that personality a voice. Then a dialogue can begin, followed by movement to a "better" place and hence a resolution that enables the condition to leave. That might require an ancestor being brought in to take responsibility or for something that was hidden being revealed, acknowledged and honoured or even a combination of both.

Allow metaphors in. They are very helpful to start the ball rolling especially with a group of clients that are 1) experiencing constellations for the first time and 2) are reluctant to express themselves in connection with others for fear of disturbing family loyalties. It is always worth pointing out that whilst it is excellent to be loyal to the strengths within our role models, it is simply stupid to be loyal to bad stuff, or stuff that harms us. Most people get that.

Always pay attention to the maternal side as more important. Mitochondrial DNA is passed through the generations. My mitochondrial DNA was formed in my grandmother's womb half way through the pregnancy that produced my mother in 1915 – over a hundred years ago now!

So what are we looking for in a constellation on health, mental or physical or emotional? What does the illness perform as a way of supporting the system albeit erroneously? What does the illness hide from clear view about the system? Do we have permission to look?

That will give us the guidelines for what representatives we need to start the ball rolling. Having established the start point it is often helpful to just watch where the representatives move to. It's like water moving downhill – it is inevitable that the constellation will find its equilibrium. Personally, when I facilitate such pieces of work I am quite bold in suggesting possible representatives, because as said before if they are superfluous they can sit down again, whereas they might just show a key to a new doorway that hadn't been seen before, as with the rotting meat smell triggering a whole other story.

It is perfectly in order to mix up constellations with people and concepts or aspects, so you might have representatives for the client, the grandma, cancer and the secret. Gradually it becomes clear that cancer hides the secret and hence the secret becomes associated with the cancer, releasing the client from her association with the cancer. At that point grandma changes her countenance and it becomes clear that the secret belongs to her and it ceases to be relevant that there even is a secret. The cancer then becomes less important in the constellation and recedes – hopefully followed in real life by that same energy – the cancer loses its grip on the client and recedes.

It sounds fanciful, but it has been documented many times and although my own research is inevitably quite limited in numbers, the outcomes of constellation work has very often led to people identifying a change in a major aspect of their lives including serious health conditions being attributed to the day they did a constellation. The aspects noted have been in the physical, mental, emotional and spiritual realms.

Chapter 13 – Rituals and Ceremonies to clear ancestral timeline issues

In the constellation about the skin condition what showed up is the likely direction for the source of the original trauma that caused the skin condition to manifest. Chemicals and medicines hadn't touched the issue as it was a somatic response to an emotional issue. Treating the next bit of the constellation as a ritual observing of the next generation as superior and therefore responsible, it becomes possible to hand the issue back along the line of ancestors and it hardly matters to the client how far back it goes, or whether the original fault is re-placed, it is simply the case that the issue has been handed back towards its origin and the client is then free to cure and to heal.

In another ceremony an elderly man felt that his stuff had come from outside his own experience and was puzzled. On setting up the constellation it became clear that the grandfather had never been mourned. Indeed, there appeared to never have been a funeral. At that point the client revealed that his grandfather had died a pauper in the workhouse. A large stone was chosen to represent the grandfather and a burial ceremony was carried out. The grief shown by the participants attending a mock up event some hundred years after the fact had to be seen to be believed. It was exactly as though they had attended a genuine funeral of the client's grandfather.

In another piece of work, it became clear that a system of parenting the parents had been established so that responsibilities always lay in the wrong direction – it has to be seen that without you parents you wouldn't exist – not the other way round. The ritual establish for supporting the work that had been done in constellation was simply to print out some photos with grandparents placed at the back, with parents in front of them facing out and then children and then at the very front, grandchildren. This was to be acknowledged by the statement "I take my place" said daily by the client towards the photos thus reinforcing that she had no responsibility for her mother and that her mother had no responsibility for her mother and so on. It enabled the client to resolve a long term anxiety and fear that as soon as her mother was not being attended to, something dreadful would befall her. I have used the photo sequence on a number of occasions to reinforce work that has been done in constellations where a dependent line has been facing backwards. In those scenarios children get ignored and abused, so it is pretty important to establish correct lines of responsibility.

Chapter 14 – Conclusion

Constellations enable us to see how the energies of the family system get passed down the generations. Sometimes we find that there are things in our lives that just won't fit, or don't belong. Constellations show us how and where they fit. They are not a quick fix for all issues of health and wellbeing and they do not need to be exaggerated in their effects. They are very good at starting the process of unravelling MSP events in our history.

Health constellations are run like any other constellation. It starts with a conversation with the client exactly when he or she is ready to work. The conversation yields the building blocks of the constellation – who are the participants and what, if any, other aspects are required to assist the process. If there appears to be a dynamic as soon as the system is setup, personally, I would let it run itself. If not, then I would inquire of the representatives what they are experiencing standing in the place of whoever or whatever they are there to represent.

As the constellation unfolds, various aspects change and evolve so that by the end of the piece of work a number of energies that proved to be difficult for the client to manage within his or her life have found a new place and the energies are now much easier to handle. The healing has begun. If the health issue is physical or mental, then any medication must under all circumstances be maintained according to the medical adviser's guidelines. However, over time it may become clear that the symptoms of the somatic experience are evolving or dissipating (somatic is when emotional pain is expressed in the physical realm as real pain or illness). At that point curing and healing will have begun to coexist within the client.

For further information, see

http://www.rafenauen.com

or call 01332 232756

or email rafe@rafenauen.com

Other books are available by searching for Rafe Nauen in Amazon (There is only one Rafe Nauen in the world and it's me) or going to http://books.rafenauen.com